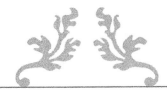

THE ESSENTIAL RENAL DIET COOKBOOK

50 Simple Low Sodium And Low Potassium Recipes To Live An Healthy Lifestyle

Sarah Gessele

© **Copyright 2021 - All rights reserved.**

The content contained within this book may not be reproduced, duplicated or transmitted without direct written permission from the author or the publisher.

Under no circumstances will any blame or legal responsibility be held against the publisher, or author, for any damages, reparation, or monetary loss due to the information contained within this book. Either directly or indirectly.

Legal Notice:

This book is copyright protected. This book is only for personal use. You cannot amend, distribute, sell, use, quote or paraphrase any part, or the content within this book, without the consent of the author or publisher.

Disclaimer Notice:

Please note the information contained within this document is for educational and entertainment purposes only. All effort has been executed to present accurate, up to date, and reliable, complete information. No warranties of any kind are declared or implied. Readers acknowledge that the author is not engaging in the rendering of legal, financial, medical or professional advice. The content within this book has been derived from various sources. Please consult a licensed professional before attempting any techniques outlined in this book.

By reading this document, the reader agrees that under no circumstances is the author responsible for any losses, direct or indirect, which are incurred as a result of the use of information contained within this document, including, but not limited to, errors, omissions, or inaccuracies.

Table of Contents

INTRODUCTION 9

BREAKFAST 12

    1. Cilantro Lime Salmon 12

    2. Asian Ginger tuna 14

    3. Cheesy Tuna Chowder 16

    4. Marinated Salmon Steak 18

    5. Tuna with honey Glaze 20

    6. Stuffed Mushrooms 21

    7. Easy Salmon and Brussels sprouts 23

    8. Salmon in Dill Sauce 24

    9. Shrimp Lo Mein 25

    10. Salmon and Carrots Mix 27

    11. Smoked Salmon and Radishes 28

    12. Parmesan Baked Fish 29

    13. Shrimp and Mango Mix 30

    14. Roasted hake 31

    15. Eggs Benedict 32

    16. Cranberry and Apple Oatmeal 34

    17. Blueberry Breakfast Smoothie 36

LUNCH 39

    18. Zucchini Bowl 39

    19. Nice Coconut Haddock 41

    20. Vegetable Rice Casserole 42

    21. Kidney Disease Stage 1 44

    22. Zucchini Garlic Fries 46

- 23. Mashed Cauliflower 47
- 24. Stir-Fried Eggplant 48
- 25. Sautéed Garlic Mushrooms 49
- 26. Stir-Fried Asparagus and Bell Pepper 50
- 27. Wild Rice with Spicy Chickpeas 51
- 28. Cashew Pesto & Parsley with veggies 53

DINNER 56
- 29. Chicken salad balsamic 56
- 30. Chicken salad with apples, grapes, and walnuts 57
- 31. Chicken strawberry green lettuce salad with ginger-lime dressing 58
- 32. Asian chicken satay 60

POULTRY 62
- 33. Chicken Veronique 62
- 34. Chicken and Apple Curry 64
- 35. London Broil 66
- 36. Sirloin with Squash and Pineapple 67
- 37. Slow-Cooked BBQ Beef 69
- 38. Lemon Sprouts 70
- 39. Lemon and Broccoli Platter 71
- 40. Chicken Liver Stew 72
- 41. Simple Lamb Chops 73
- 42. Chicken and Mushroom Stew 74

SNACKS 76
- 43. Hummus Deviled Eggs 77
- 44. Hummus with Celery 78
- 45. Lemony Ginger Cookies 80
- 46. Mandarin Cottage Cheese 82

| | 47. | Mushroom Chips | 83 |

DESSERTS 85

	48.	Pound Cake with Pineapple	86
	49.	Apple Crunch Pie	88
	50.	Vanilla Custard	89
	51.	Chocolate Chip Cookies	90

INTRODUCTION

The renal diet has been in use since the middle of the 20th century when the popular scientist discovered some thoughts and conclusions that were healthy and useful for the renal diet. The diet has also improved the health of kidney patients, but it also helps to avoid complications with the kidneys.

Your intake of sodium, protein, potassium and phosphorus is regulated by the Renal Diet. The prevention of renal failure is aided by a renal diet. This is a list of foods/nutrients that should be avoided to prevent kidney problems:

Phosphate: When kidney failure approaches 80 percent and goes to the 4th/5th level of kidney failure, phosphate intake becomes risky. So, by counting the calories and minerals, it is easier to lower your phosphate intake.

Potassium: If your results indicate that your potassium level is elevated in the blood after being diagnosed, then you can reduce your potassium intake. Carrots that are baked and fried are very rich in potassium. Leafy greens, with high levels of potassium in fruit juices. Vegetables low in potassium can still be enjoyed.

Sodium: In our diet, adding salt is very important, but you have to omit or minimize your salt intake when you are suffering from kidney problems. High blood pressure and fluid accumulation in the body can be caused by too much sodium intake. You need to find alternatives that will help season your food. A good choice is herbs and spices that are extracted from plants. Without adding any salt, using garlic, pepper and mustard will improve the taste of your food. Stop sodium-low artificial "salts" because they are rich in potassium, which is also harmful for kidney health.

This cookbook's recipes are plain, tasty, and nutritious. You can also use them to experiment and build your renal diet recipes as an inspiration. It is also possible to see these samples as snacks for you during the day.

A low sodium diet is provided in this cookbook, so knowing the reason for sodium intake is important. Through adding potassium, low sodium consumption, and adding fiber, a low sodium renal diet can be achieved. Many individuals fail to add extra fiber to the diet, and it is viewed as an unhealthy factor many times. But you will soon appreciate the advantages when applied to the renal diet.

You should work with the recipes from this cookbook if you're still used to the renal diet. For more serious and vigilant renal diet beginners, you may use the guide. Try these fast recipes for a better taste if you want to live a happy, safe renal diet!

BREAKFAST

1. Cilantro Lime Salmon

Preparation Time: 10 min

Cooking Time: 20 minutes

Servings: 4

Ingredients:

- ¼ cup olive oil
- ¼ cup chopped fresh cilantro
- ½ teaspoon chopped garlic
- 5 (5 ounce) fillets salmon
- Ground black pepper to taste
- ½ lemon, juiced
- ½ lime, juiced

Directions:
1. Heat the olive oil in a skillet over medium heat.
2. Stir cilantro and garlic into the oil; cook about 1 minute.
3. Season salmon fillets with black pepper; lay gently into the oil mixture.
4. Place a cover on the skillet. Cook fillets 10 minutes, turn, and continue cooking until the fish flakes easily with a fork and is lightly browned, about 10 minutes more.
5. Squeeze lemon juice and lime juice over the fillets to serve.

Nutrition: Calories 249, Total Fat 18.7g, Saturated Fat 3.3g, Cholesterol 18mg, Sodium 48mg, Total Carbohydrate 1.7g, Dietary Fiber 0.5g, Total Sugars 0.3g, Protein 20.7g, Calcium 6mg, Iron 0mg, Potassium 26mg, Phosphorus 20 mg

2. Asian Ginger tuna

Preparation Time: 10 min

Cooking Time: 20 minutes

Servings: 4

Ingredients:

- 1 cup water
- 1 tablespoon minced fresh ginger root
- 1 tablespoon minced garlic
- 2 tablespoons soy sauce
- 1 1/4 pounds thin tuna fillets
- 6 large white mushrooms, sliced
- 1/4 cup sliced green onion
- 1 tablespoon chopped fresh cilantro (optional)

Directions:
1. Put water, ginger, and garlic in a wide pot with a lid.
2. Bring the water to a boil, reduce heat to medium-low, and simmer 3 to 5 minutes.
3. Stir soy sauce into the water mixture; add tuna fillets.
4. Place cover on the pot, bring water to a boil, and let cook for 3 minutes more.
5. Add mushrooms, cover, and cook until the fish loses pinkness and begins to flake, about 3 minutes more.
6. Sprinkle green onion over the fillets, cover, and cook for 30 seconds.
7. Garnish with cilantro to serve.

Nutrition: Calories 109, Total Fat 7.9g, Saturated Fat 0g, Cholesterol 0mg, Sodium 454mg, Total Carbohydrate 3.1g, Dietary Fiber 0.6g, Total Sugars 0.9g, Protein 7.1g, Calcium 10mg, Iron 1mg, Potassium 158mg, Phosphorus 120 mg

3. Cheesy Tuna Chowder

Preparation Time: 10 min

Cooking Time: 20 minutes

Servings: 4

Ingredients:

- 2 tablespoons olive oil
- 1/2 small onion, chopped
- 1 cup water
- 1/2 cup chopped celery
- 1 cup sliced baby carrots
- 3 cups soy almond milk, divided
- 1/3 cup all-purpose flour
- 1/2 teaspoon ground black pepper
- 1 1/2 pounds tuna fillets, cut into 1-inch pieces
- 1 1/2 cups shredded Cheddar cheese

Directions:

1. In a Dutch oven over medium heat, heat olive oil and sauté the onion until tender. Pour in water. Mix in celery, carrots, cook 10 minutes, stirring occasionally, until vegetables are tender.
2. In a small bowl, whisk together 1 1/2 cups almond milk and all-purpose flour. Mix into the Dutch oven.

3. Mix remaining almond milk, and pepper into the Dutch oven. Stirring occasionally, continue cooking the mixture about 10 minutes, until thickened.
4. Stir tuna into the mixture, and cook 5 minutes, or until fish is easily flaked with a fork. Mix in Cheddar cheese, and cook another 5 minutes, until melted.

Nutrition: Calories 228, Total Fat 15.5g, Saturated Fat 6.5g, Cholesterol 30mg, Sodium 206mg, Total Carbohydrate 10.8g, Dietary Fiber 1g, Total Sugars 4.1g, Protein 11.6g, Calcium 183mg, Iron 1mg, Potassium 163mg, Phosphorus 150 mg

4. Marinated Salmon Steak

Preparation Time: 10 min

Cooking Time: 10 minutes

Servings: 4

Ingredients:

- ¼ cup lime juice
- ¼ cup soy sauce
- 2 tablespoons olive oil
- 1 tablespoon lemon juice
- 2 tablespoons chopped fresh parsley
- 1 clove garlic, minced
- ½ teaspoon chopped fresh oregano
- ½ teaspoon ground black pepper
- 4 (4 ounce) salmon steaks

Directions:

1. In a large non-reactive dish, mix together the lime juice, soy sauce, olive oil, lemon juice, parsley, garlic, oregano, and pepper. Place the salmon steaks in the marinade and turn to coat. Cover, and refrigerate for at least 30 minutes.
2. Preheat grill for high heat.
3. Lightly oil grill grate. Cook the salmon steaks for 5 to 6 minutes, then salmon and baste with the marinade. Cook for an additional 5 minutes, or to desired doneness. Discard any remaining marinade.

Nutrition: Calories 108, Total Fat 8.4g, Saturated Fat 1.2g, Cholesterol 9mg, Sodium 910mg, Total Carbohydrate 3.6g, Dietary Fiber 0.4g, Total Sugars 1.7g, Protein 5.4g, Calcium 19mg, Iron 1mg, Potassium 172mg, Phosphorus 165 mg

5. Tuna with honey Glaze

Preparation Time: 10 min

Cooking Time: 10 minutes

Servings: 4

Ingredients:

- 1/4 cup honey
- 2 tablespoons Dijon mustard
- 4 (6 ounce) boneless tuna fillets
- Ground black pepper to taste

Directions:

1. Preheat the oven's broiler and set the oven rack at about 6 inches from the heat source; prepare the rack of a broiler pan with cooking spray.
2. Season the tuna with pepper and arrange onto the prepared broiler pan. Whisk together the honey and Dijon mustard in a small bowl; spoon mixture evenly onto top of salmon fillets.
3. Cook under the preheated broiler until the fish flakes easily with a fork, 10 to 15 minutes.

Nutrition: Calories 160, Total Fat 8.1g, Saturated Fat 0g, Cholesterol 0mg, Sodium 90mg, Total Carbohydrate 17.9g, Dietary Fiber 0.3g, Total Sugars 17.5g, Protein 5.7g, Calcium 6mg, Iron 0mg, Potassium 22mg, Phosphorus 16 mg

6. Stuffed Mushrooms

Preparation Time: 10 min

Cooking Time: 10 minutes

Servings: 4

Ingredients:

- 12 large fresh mushrooms, stems removed
- ½ pound crabmeat, flaked
- 2 cups olive oil
- 2 cloves garlic, peeled and minced
- Garlic powder to taste
- Crushed red pepper to taste

Directions:
1. Arrange mushroom caps on a medium baking sheet, bottoms up. Chop and reserve mushroom stems.
2. Preheat oven to 350 degrees F.
3. In a medium saucepan over medium heat, heat oil. Mix in garlic and cook until tender, about 5 minutes.
4. In a medium bowl, mix together reserved mushroom stems, and crab meat. Liberally stuff mushrooms with the mixture. Drizzle with the garlic. Season with garlic powder and crushed red pepper.
5. Bake uncovered in the preheated oven 10 to 12 minutes, or until stuffing is lightly browned.

Nutrition: Calories 312, Total Fat 33.8g, Saturated Fat 4.8g, Cholesterol 4mg, Sodium 160mg, Total Carbohydrate 3.8g, Dietary Fiber 0.3g, Total Sugars 1.6g, Protein 2.2g, Calcium 3mg, Iron 1mg, Potassium 93mg, Phosphorus 86 mg

7. Easy Salmon and Brussels sprouts

Preparation Time: 10 minutes

Cooking Time: 10 minutes

Servings: 6

Ingredients:

- 6 deboned medium salmon fillets
- 1 tsp. onion powder
- 1 ¼ lbs. halved Brussels sprouts
- 3 tbsps. Extra virgin extra virgin olive oil
- 2 tbsps. Brown sugar
- 1 tsp. garlic powder
- 1 tsp. smoked paprika

Directions:

1. In a bowl, mix sugar with onion powder, garlic powder, smoked paprika as well as a number of tablespoon olive oil and whisk well.
2. Spread Brussels sprouts about the lined baking sheet, drizzle the rest in the essential extra virgin olive oil, toss to coat, introduce in the oven at 450 0F and bake for 5 minutes.
3. Add salmon fillets brush with sugar mix you've prepared, introduce inside the oven and bake for 15 minutes more.
4. Divide everything between plates and serve.
5. Enjoy!

Nutrition: Calories: 212, Fat: 5 g, Carbs: 12 g, Protein: 8 g, Sugars: 3.7 g, Sodium: 299.1 mg

8. Salmon in Dill Sauce

Preparation Time: 10 minutes

Cooking Time: 10 minutes

Servings: 6

Ingredients:

- 6 salmon fillets
- 1 c. low-fat, low-sodium chicken broth
- 1 tsp. cayenne pepper
- 2 tbsps. Fresh lemon juice
- 2 c. water
- ¼ c. chopped fresh dill

Directions:

1. In a slow cooker, mix together water, broth, lemon juice, lemon juice and dill.
2. Arrange salmon fillets on top, skin side down.
3. Sprinkle with cayenne pepper.
4. Set the slow cooker on low.
5. Cover and cook for about 1-2 hours.

Nutrition: Calories: 360, Fat: 8 g, Carbs: 44 g, Protein: 28 g, Sugars: 0.5 g, Sodium: 8 mg

9. Shrimp Lo Mein

Preparation Time: 10 minutes

Cooking Time: 10 minutes

Servings: 6

Ingredients:

- 1 tbsp. cornstarch
- 1 lb. medium-size frozen raw shrimp
- 1 c. frozen shelled edamame
- 3 tbsps. Light teriyaki sauce
- 16 0z. Drained and rinsed tofu spaghetti noodles
- 18 oz. frozen Szechuan vegetable blend with sesame sauce

Directions:
1. Microwave noodles for 1 minute; set aside. Place shrimp in a small bowl and toss with 2 tablespoons teriyaki sauce; set aside.
2. Place mixed vegetables and edamame in a large nonstick skillet with 1/4 cup water. Cover and cook, stirring occasionally, over medium-high heat for 7 minutes or until cooked through.
3. Stir shrimp into vegetable mixture; cover and cook 4 to 5 minutes or until shrimp is pink and cooked through.
4. Stir together remaining 1 tablespoon teriyaki sauce and the cornstarch, then stir into the mixture in the skillet until thickened. Gently stir noodles into skillet and cook until warmed through.

Nutrition: Calories: 252, Fat: 7.1 g, Carbs: 35.2 g, Protein: 12.1 g, Sugars: 2.2 g, Sodium: 180 mg

10. Salmon and Carrots Mix

Preparation Time: 10 minutes

Cooking Time: 10 minutes

Servings: 4

Ingredients:

- 4 oz. chopped smoked salmon
- 1 tbsp. essential olive oil
- Black pepper
- 1 tbsp. chopped chives
- ¼ c. coconut cream
- 1 ½ lbs. chopped carrots
- 2 tsps. Prepared horseradish

Directions:

1. Heat up a pan using the oil over medium heat, add carrots and cook for 10 minutes.
2. Add salmon, chives, horseradish, cream and black pepper, toss, cook for 1 minute more, divide between plates and serve.
3. Enjoy!

Nutrition: Calories: 233, Fat: 6 g, Carbs: 9 g, Protein: 11 g, Sugars: 3.3 g, Sodium: 97 mg

11. Smoked Salmon and Radishes

Preparation Time: 10 minutes

Cooking Time: 10 minutes

Servings: 8

Ingredients:

- ½ c. drained and chopped capers
- 1 lb. skinless, de-boned and flaked smoked salmon
- 4 chopped radishes
- 3 tbsps. Chopped chives
- 3 tbsps. Prepared beet horseradish
- 2 tsps. Grated lemon zest
- 1/3 c. roughly chopped red onion

Directions:

1. In a bowl, combine the salmon while using the beet horseradish, lemon zest, radish, capers, onions and chives, toss and serve cold.
2. Enjoy!

Nutrition: Calories: 254, Fat: 2 g, Carbs: 7 g, Protein: 7 g, Sugars: 1.4 g, Sodium: 660 mg

12. Parmesan Baked Fish

Preparation Time: 10 minutes

Cooking Time: 10 minutes

Servings: 4

Ingredients:

- ½ tsp. Worcestershire sauce
- 1/3 c. mayonnaise
- 3 tbsps. Freshly grated parmesan cheese
- 4 oz. cod fish fillets
- 1 tbsp. snipped fresh chives

Directions:

1. Preheat oven to 450°C.
2. Rinse fish and pat dry with paper towels; spray an 8x8x2" baking dish with non-stick pan spray, set aside.
3. In small bowl stir mayo, grated cheese, chives, and Worcestershire sauce; spread mixture over fish fillets.
4. Bake, uncovered, 12-15 minutes or until fish flakes easily with a fork

Nutrition: Calories: 850.5, Fat: 24.8g, Carbs: 44.5 g, Protein: 104.6 g, Sugars: 0.6 g, Sodium: 307.7 mg

13. Shrimp and Mango Mix

Preparation Time: 10 minutes

Cooking Time: 10 minutes

Servings: 4

Ingredients:

- 3 tbsps. Finely chopped parsley
- 3 tbsps. Coconut sugar
- 1 lb. peeled, deveined and cooked shrimp
- 3 tbsps. Balsamic vinegar
- 3 peeled and cubed mangos

Directions:

1. In a bowl, mix vinegar with sugar and mayo and whisk.
2. In another bowl, combine the mango with the parsley and shrimp, add the mayo mix, toss and serve.
3. Enjoy!

Nutrition: Calories: 204, Fat: 3 g, Carbs: 8 g, Protein: 8 g, Sugars: 12.6 g, Sodium: 273.4 mg

14. Roasted hake

Preparation Time: 20 minutes

Cooking Time: 30 minutes

Servings: 4

Ingredients:

- ½ c. tomato sauce
- 2 sliced Red bell peppers
- Fresh parsley
- ½ c. grated cheese
- 4 lbs. deboned hake fish
- 1 tbsp. olive oil
- Salt.

Directions:

1. Season the fish with salt. Pan-fry the fish until half-done.
2. Shape foil into containers according to the number of fish pieces.
3. Pour tomato sauce into each foil dish; arrange the fish, then the tomato slices, again add tomato sauce and sprinkle with grated cheese.
4. Bake in the oven at 400 F until there is a golden crust.
5. Serve with fresh parsley.

Nutrition: Calories: 421, Fat: 48.7 g, Carbs: 2.4 g, Protein: 17.4 g, Sugars: 0.5 g, Sodium: 94.6 mg

15. Eggs Benedict

Preparation Time: 20 minutes

Cooking Time: 35 Minutes

Servings: 4

Ingredients:

- 2 pieces of toasted bread - white flour
- 4 eggs
- 3 egg yolks
- 1 tablespoon lemon juice
- ½ teaspoon of cayenne pepper
- ½ teaspoon of paprika
- 1 tablespoon apple cider vinegar
- 2 tablespoons of unsalted butter

Direction:

1. Slice the two toasted bread pieces in two, so you can end up with four pieces where each piece represents one serving.
2. Take a large skillet or a pot and pour one cup of water in it. Add a tablespoon of vinegar and bring the water to boil. When the water starts to boil, break four eggs, one at the time, and poach the eggs by covering the skillet. Eggs should be done between 3 and 5 minutes of poaching, depending on how you like your eggs cooked.
3. Next place poached eggs on top of bread pieces. Take a skillet and add the butter to melt it then add cayenne and paprika to

the melted butter. Beat the egg yolks over medium heat then add the eggs to the mixture with butter. Add lemon juice and whisk it into the egg and butter mixture. Once the sauce reaches an adequate thickness, remove from the heat and pour over the eggs and toasted bread.

Nutrition: Potassium 146 mg Sodium 206 mg Phosphorus 114 mg Calories 316

16. Cranberry and Apple Oatmeal

Preparation Time: 10 minutes

Cooking Time: 25 Minutes

Servings: 2

Ingredients:

- 1 apple – diced
- ¼ teaspoon nutmeg
- ¼ cup cranberry – fresh
- 2/3 cup oatmeal – you can use quick oatmeal with no added sodium and extra potassium – avoid whole grain if not on dialysis
- ½ teaspoon cinnamon
- 2 cup water

Direction:

1. You need to prepare all the ingredients and cut the apple in small pieces. Pour two cups of water into a saucepan and add the diced apple, cranberries, nutmeg and cinnamon.
2. Seal the saucepan and bring the water with ingredients to boil. Cook until the fruit is tender, which shouldn't take more than 5 to 10 minutes.
3. Check if apples are tender then add 2/3 cup oatmeal to the boiling water. Stir in and cook for around one minute before serving the oatmeal. Based on your doctor's recommendations you can serve the oatmeal with an adequate dose of milk or add milk substitute to the oatmeal when serving.

Nutrition: Potassium 170 mg Sodium 59 mg Phosphorus 187 mg Calories 173

17. Blueberry Breakfast Smoothie

Preparation Time: 10 minutes

Cooking Time: 10 Minutes

Servings: 1

Ingredients:

- 1/3 cup vanilla almond milk – no sugar added
- 2 tablespoons protein powder of your choice
- ¼ cup of Greek yogurt - look for brands with low sodium and low potassium
- 3 strawberries - fresh, sliced
- 6 raspberries
- 1 cup blueberries – frozen or fresh
- 1 tablespoon cereal – avoid whole grain due to high levels of potassium

Direction:

1. First, you need to blend one cup of blueberries in a food processor, blending the fruit on low speed for around a minute.
2. After a minute, add almond milk, protein powder and Greek yogurt to blended blueberries and blend the mixture for another minute or until the blueberry smoothie turns into a homogeneous mass.
3. Pour the smoothie in a bowl, add cereals, raspberries, sliced strawberries, and serve.

Nutrition: Potassium 270 mg Sodium 108 mg Phosphorus 114 mg Calories 225

LUNCH

18. Zucchini Bowl

Preparation Time: 10 minutes

Cooking Time: 20 minutes

Servings: 4

Ingredients:

- 1 onion, chopped
- 3 zucchini, cut into medium chunks
- 2 tablespoons coconut almond milk
- 2 garlic cloves, minced
- 4 cups chicken stock
- 2 tablespoons coconut oil
- Pinch of salt
- Black pepper to taste

Directions:
1. Take a pot and place it over medium heat
2. Add oil and let it heat up
3. Add zucchini, garlic, onion, and stir
4. Cook for 5 minutes
5. Add stock, salt, pepper, and stir
6. Bring to a boil and lower down the heat
7. Simmer for 20 minutes.
8. Remove heat and add coconut almond milk
9. Use an immersion blender until smooth
10. Ladle into soup bowls and serve
11. Enjoy!

Nutrition: Calories: 160 Fat: 2g Carbohydrates: 4g Protein: 7g

19. Nice Coconut Haddock

Preparation Time: 10 minutes

Cooking Time: 12 minutes

Servings: 3

Ingredients:

- 4 haddock fillets, 5 ounces each, boneless
- 2 tablespoons coconut oil, melted
- 1 cup coconut, shredded and unsweetened
- ¼ cup hazelnuts, ground
- Salt to taste

Directions:

1. Preheat your oven to 400 °F
2. Line a baking sheet with parchment paper
3. Keep it on the side
4. Pat fish fillets with a paper towel and season with salt
5. Take a bowl and stir in hazelnuts and shredded coconut
6. Drag fish fillets through the coconut mix until both sides are coated well
7. Transfer to a baking dish
8. Brush with coconut oil
9. Bake for about 12 minutes until flaky
10. Serve and enjoy!

Nutrition: Calories: 299 Fat: 24g Carbohydrates: 1g Protein: 20g

20. Vegetable Rice Casserole

Preparation Time: 10 minutes

Cooking Time: 50 minutes

Servings: 4

Ingredients:

- 1 teaspoon of olive oil
- ½ small sweet onion, chopped
- ½ teaspoon of minced garlic
- ½ cup of chopped red bell pepper
- ¼ cup of grated carrot
- 1 cup of white basmati rice
- 2 cups of water
- ¼ cup of grated Parmesan cheese
- Freshly ground black pepper

Directions:

1. Preheat the oven to 350°f.
2. In a medium skillet over medium-high heat, heat the olive oil.
3. Add the onion and garlic, and sauté until softened, about 3 minutes.
4. Transfer the vegetables to a 9-by-9-inch baking dish, and stir in the rice and water.
5. Cover the dish and bake until the liquid is absorbed 35 to 40 minutes.

6. Sprinkle the cheese on top and bake an additional 5 minutes to melt.
7. Season the casserole with pepper, and serve.
8. Substitution tip: Not surprisingly, the cheesy topping on this casserole elevates it to a truly sublime experience. You can also try feta, Cheddar cheese, and goat cheese for different tastes and textures.

Nutrition: Calories: 224 Total fat: 3g Saturated fat: 1g Cholesterol: 6mg Sodium: 105mg Carbohydrates: 41g Fiber: 2g Phosphorus: 118mg Potassium: 176mg Protein: 6g

21. Kidney Disease Stage 1

Collard Green Wrap

Preparation Time: 10 minutes

Cooking Time: 0 minutes

Servings: 4

Ingredients:

- ½ block feta, cut into 4 (1-inch thick) strips (4-oz)
- ½ cup purple onion, diced
- ½ medium red bell pepper, julienned
- 1 medium cucumber, julienned
- 4 large cherry bell pepper, halved
- 4 large collard green leaves, washed
- 8 whole kalamata capers, halved
- Sauce Ingredients:
- 1 cup low-fat plain Greek yogurt
- 1 tablespoon white vinegar
- 1 teaspoon garlic powder
- 2 tablespoons minced fresh dill
- 2 tablespoons olive oil
- 2.5-ounces cucumber, seeded and grated (¼-whole)
- Salt and pepper to taste

Directions:

1. Make the sauce first: make sure to squeeze out all the excess liquid from the cucumber after grating. In a small bowl, put

all together the sauce ingredients and mix thoroughly then refrigerate.

2. Prepare and slice all wrap ingredients.
3. On a flat surface, spread one collard green leaf. Spread 2 tablespoons of Tzatziki sauce in the middle of the leaf.
4. Layer ¼ of each of the bell pepper, feta, capers, onion, pepper, and cucumber. Place them on the center of the leaf, like piling them high instead of spreading them.
5. Fold the leaf-like you would a burrito. Repeat process for remaining ingredients.
6. Serve and enjoy.

Nutrition: Calories 463 Fat 31g Carbs 31g Protein 20g Fiber 7g

22. Zucchini Garlic Fries

Preparation Time: 10 minutes

Cooking Time: 20 minutes

Servings: 6

Ingredients:

- ¼ teaspoon garlic powder
- ½ cup almond flour
- 2 large egg whites, beaten
- 3 medium zucchinis, sliced into fry sticks
- Salt and pepper to taste

Directions:

1. Set the oven to 400F.
2. Mix all together the ingredients in a bowl until the zucchini fries are well coated.
3. Place fries on the cookie sheet and spread evenly.
4. Put in the oven and cook for 20 minutes.
5. Halfway through cooking time, stir-fries.

Nutrition: Calories 11 Fat 0.1g, Carbs 1g Protein1.5 g Fiber 0.5g

23. Mashed Cauliflower

Preparation Time: 10 minutes

Cooking Time: 10 minutes

Servings: 3

Ingredients:

- 1 cauliflower head
- 1 tablespoon olive oil
- ½ tsp salt
- ¼ tsp dill
- Pepper to taste
- 2 tbsp. low-fat almond milk

Directions:

1. Place a small pot of water to a boil.
2. Chop cauliflower in florets.
3. Add florets to boiling water and boil uncovered for 5 minutes. Turn off fire and let it sit for 5 minutes more.
4. In a blender, add all ingredients except for cauliflower and blend to mix well.
5. Drain cauliflower well and add it to a blender. Puree until smooth and creamy.
6. Serve and enjoy.

Nutrition: Calories 78 Fat 5g Carbs 6g Protein 2g Fiber 2g

24. Stir-Fried Eggplant

Preparation Time: 10 minutes

Cooking Time: 10 minutes

Servings: 2

Ingredients:

- 1 tablespoon coconut oil
- 2 eggplants, sliced into 3-inch in length
- 4 cloves of garlic, minced
- 1 onion, chopped
- 1 teaspoon ginger, grated
- 1 teaspoon lemon juice, freshly squeezed
- ½ tsp salt
- ½ tsp pepper

Directions:

1. Heat oil in a nonstick saucepan.
2. Pan-fry the eggplants for 2 minutes on all sides.
3. Add the garlic and onions until fragrant, around 3 minutes.
4. Stir in the ginger, salt, pepper, and lemon juice.
5. Add a ½ cup of water and bring to a simmer. Cook until eggplant is tender.

Nutrition: Calories 232 Fat 8g Carbs 41g Protein 7g Fiber 18g

25. Sautéed Garlic Mushrooms

Preparation Time: 10 minutes

Cooking Time: 10 minutes

Servings: 4

Ingredients:

- 1 tablespoon olive oil
- 3 cloves of garlic, minced
- 16 ounces fresh brown mushrooms, sliced
- 7 ounces fresh shiitake mushrooms, sliced
- ½ tsp salt
- ½ tsp pepper or more to taste

Directions:

1. Place a nonstick saucepan on medium-high fire and heat pan for a minute.
2. Add oil and heat for 2 minutes.
3. Stir in garlic and sauté for a minute.
4. Add remaining ingredients and stir fry until soft and tender, around 5 minutes.
5. Turn off fire, let mushrooms rest while the pan is covered for 5 minutes.
6. Serve and enjoy.

Nutrition: Calories 95 Fat 4g Carbs 14g Protein 3g, Fiber 4g

26. Stir-Fried Asparagus and Bell Pepper

Preparation Time: 10 minutes

Cooking Time: 10 minutes

Servings: 6

Ingredients:

- 1 tablespoon olive oil
- 4 cloves of garlic, minced
- 1-pound fresh asparagus spears, trimmed
- 2 large red bell peppers, seeded and julienned
- ½ teaspoon thyme
- 5 tablespoons water
- ½ tsp salt
- ½ tsp pepper or more to taste

Directions:

1. Place a nonstick saucepan on high fire and heat pan for a minute.
2. Add oil and heat for 2 minutes.
3. Stir in garlic and sauté for a minute.
4. Add remaining ingredients and stir fry until soft and tender, around 6 minutes.
5. Turn off fire, let veggies rest while the pan is covered for 5 minutes.

Nutrition: Calories 45 Fat 2g Carbs 5g, Net Protein 2g Fiber 2g

27. Wild Rice with Spicy Chickpeas

Preparation Time: 15 minutes

Cooking Time: 60 minutes

Servings: 6-7

Ingredients:

- 1 Cup basmati rice
- 1 Cup wild rice
- Salt & pepper to taste
- 4tbsp Olive oil
- 1tbsp Garlic powder
- 2tsp cumin powder
- ¼ Cup sunflower oil
- 3 Cups chickpeas
- 1tsp Flour
- 1tsp Curry powder
- 3tsp Paprika powder
- 1tsp Dill
- 3tbsp parsley (chopped)
- 1 Medium onion (thinly sliced)
- 2 Cups currants

Directions:

1. For cooking wild rice, fill the half pot with water and bring it to boil. Put the rice and let it simmer for at least 40 minutes.

2. Take olive in the pot and heat it on medium flame. Now add cumin powder, salt, and water and bring it to boil. Then add basmati rice and cook for 20 minutes.
3. Leave rice for cooking and prepare spicy chickpeas. Heat 2tbsp of olive oil in the pan and toss chickpeas, garlic powder, salt & pepper, cumin, and paprika powder in it.
4. In another pan, cook onion with sunflower oil until it is golden brown and add flour.
5. Mix flour and onion with your hands.
6. For serving, place both types of rice in a bowl with spicy chickpeas and fry the onion. Garnish it with parsley and herbs.

Nutrition: Calories: 647 kcal Protein: 25.43 g Fat: 25.72 g Carbohydrates: 88.3 g

28. Cashew Pesto & Parsley with veggies

Preparation Time: 15 minutes

Cooking Time: 10 minutes

Servings: 3-4

Ingredients:

- 3 Zucchini (sliced)
- 8 Soaked bamboo skewers
- 2 Red capsicums
- ¼Cup olive oil
- 750grams Eggplant
- 4 Lemon cheeks
- For Serving
- Couscous salad
- For Preparing Cashew Pesto
- ½Cup cashew (roasted)
- ½ Cup parsley
- 2 Cup grated parmesan
- 2tbsp Lime juice
- ¼Cup olive oil

Directions:

1. Toss capsicum, eggplant, and zucchini with oil and salt and thread it onto skewers.
2. Cook bamboo sticks for 6-8 minutes on a barbecue grill pan on medium heat.

3. Also, grill lemon cheeks from both sides.
4. For preparing cashew pesto, combine all ingredients in the food processor and blend.
5. For serving, place grill skewers in a plate with grill lemon slices and drizzle some cashew pesto over it.

Nutrition: Calories: 666 kcal Protein: 23.96 g Fat: 48.04 g Carbohydrates: 41.4 g

DINNER

29. Chicken salad balsamic

Preparation time 15 minutes

Cooking Time: 15 minutes

Servings: 6

Ingredients

- 3 cup diced cold, cooked chicken
- 1 cup diced apple
- 1/2 cup diced celery
- 2 green onions, chopped
- 1/2 cup chopped walnuts
- 3 tablespoons. Balsamic vinegar
- 5 tablespoons. Olive oil
- Salt and pepper to taste

Directions

1. Toss together the celery, chicken, onion, walnuts, and apple in a big bowl.
2. Whisk the oil together with the vinegar in a small bowl. Pour the dressing over the salad. Then add pepper and salt to taste. Combine the ingredients thoroughly. Leave the mixture for 10-15 minutes. Toss once more and chill.

Nutrition: calories: 336 total fat: 26.8 g carbohydrates: 6g protein: 19 g cholesterol: 55 mg sodium: 58 mg

30. Chicken salad with apples, grapes, and walnuts

Preparation Time: 25 minutes

Cooking Time: 25 minutes

Servings: 12

Ingredients

- 4 cooked chicken breasts, shredded
- 2 granny smith apples, cut into small chunks
- 2cupchopped walnuts, or to taste
- 1/2 red onion, chopped
- 3 stalks celery, chopped
- 3 tablespoons. Lemon juice
- 1/2cupvanilla yogurt
- 5 tablespoons. Creamy salad dressing (such as miracle whip®)
- 5 tablespoons. Mayonnaise
- 25 seedless red grapes, halved

Directions

1. In a big bowl, toss together the shredded chicken, lemon juice, apple chunks, celery, red onion, and walnuts.
2. Get another bowl and whisk together the dressing, vanilla yogurt, and mayonnaise. Pour over the chicken mixture. Toss to coat. Fold the grapes carefully into the salad.

Nutrition: calories: 307 total fat: 22.7 g carbohydrates: 10.8g protein: 17.3 g cholesterol: 41 mg sodium: 128 mg

31. Chicken strawberry green lettuce salad with ginger-lime dressing

Preparation Time: 10 minutes

Cooking Time: 30 minutes

Servings: 2

Ingredients

- 2 teaspoons. Corn oil
- 1 skinless, boneless chicken breast half - cut into bite-size pieces
- 1/2 teaspoon garlic powder
- 1 1/2 tablespoons. Mayonnaise
- 1/2 lime, juiced
- 1/2 teaspoon ground ginger
- 2 teaspoons. Almond milk
- 2cupfresh green lettuce, stems removed
- 4 fresh strawberries, sliced
- 1 1/2 tablespoons. Slivered almonds
- Freshly ground black pepper to taste

Directions

1. In a skillet, heat oil over medium heat. Add the chicken breast and garlic powder. Cook the chicken for 10 minutes per side. When the juices run clear, remove from heat and set aside.
2. Combine the lime juice, almond milk, mayonnaise, and ginger in a bowl.

3. Place the green lettuce on serving dishes. Top with strawberries and chicken. Then sprinkle with almonds. Drizzle the salad with the dressing. Add pepper and serve.

Nutrition: calories: 242 total fat: 17.3 g carbohydrates: 7.5g protein: 15.8 g cholesterol: 40 mg sodium: 117 mg

32. Asian chicken satay

Preparation Time: 15 minutes

Cooking Time: 10 minutes

Servings: 6

Ingredients

- Juice of 2 limes
- Brown sugar – 2 tablespoons
- Minced garlic – 1 tablespoon
- Ground cumin – 2 teaspoons
- Boneless, skinless chicken breast – 12, cut into strips

Directions

1. In a bowl, stir together the cumin, garlic, brown sugar, and lime juice.
2. Add the chicken strips to the bowl and marinate in the refrigerator for 1 hour.
3. Heat the barbecue to medium-high.
4. Remove the chicken from the marinade and thread each strip onto wooden skewers that have been soaked in the water.
5. Grill the chicken for about 4 minutes per side or until the meat is cooked through but still juicy.

Nutrition: calories: 78 carb: 4g phosphorus: 116mg potassium: 108mg sodium: 100mg protein: 12g

POULTRY

33. Chicken Veronique

Preparation Time: 10 minutes

Cooking Time: 10 minutes

Servings: 4

Ingredients:

- 2 boneless skinless chicken breasts
- 1/2 shallot, chopped
- 2 tablespoons butter
- 2 tablespoons dry white wine
- 2 tablespoons chicken broth
- 1/2 cup green grapes, halved
- 1 teaspoon dried tarragon
- 1/4 cup cream

Directions:

1. Place an 8-inch skillet over medium heat and add butter to melt.
2. Sear the chicken in the melted butter until golden-brown on both sides.
3. Place the boneless chicken on a plate and set it aside.
4. Add shallot to the same skillet and stir until soft.
5. Whisk cornstarch with broth and wine in a small bowl.
6. Pour this slurry into the skillet and mix well.

7. Place the chicken in the skillet and cook it on a simmer for 6 minutes.
8. Transfer the chicken to the serving plate.
9. Add cream, tarragon, and grapes.
10. Cook for 1 minute, and then pour this sauce over the chicken.
11. Serve.

Nutrition: Calories: 306 kcal Total Fat: 18 g Saturated Fat: 0 g Cholesterol: 124 mg Sodium: 167 mg Total Carbs: 9 g

34. Chicken and Apple Curry

Preparation Time: 10 minutes

Cooking Time: 1 hour and 11 minutes

Servings: 8

Ingredients:

- 8 boneless skinless chicken breasts
- 1/4 teaspoon black pepper
- 2 medium apples, peeled, cored, and chopped
- 2 small onions, chopped
- 1 garlic clove, minced
- 3 tablespoons butter
- 1 tablespoon curry powder
- 1/2 tablespoon dried basil
- 3 tablespoons flour
- 1 cup chicken broth
- 1 cup of rice almond milk

Directions:

1. Preheat oven to 350°F.
2. Set the chicken breasts in a baking pan and sprinkle black pepper over it.
3. Place a suitably-sized saucepan over medium heat and add butter to melt.
4. Add onion, garlic, and apple, then sauté until soft.
5. Stir in basil and curry powder, and then cook for 1 minute.

6. Add flour and continue mixing for 1 minute.
7. Stir in rice almond milk and chicken broth, then stir cook for 5 minutes.
8. Pour this sauce over the chicken breasts in the baking pan.
9. Bake the chicken for 60 minutes then serve.

Nutrition: Calories: 232 kcal Total Fat: 8 g Saturated Fat: 0 g Cholesterol: 85 mg Sodium: 118 mg Total Carbs: 11 g

35. London Broil

Preparation Time: 10 minutes

Cooking Time: 5 minutes

Servings: 4

Ingredients:

- 2 pounds flank steak
- 1/4 teaspoon meat tenderizer
- 1 tablespoon sugar
- 2 tablespoons lemon juice
- 2 tablespoons soy sauce
- 1 tablespoon honey
- 1 teaspoon herb seasoning blend

Directions:

1. Pound the meat with a mallet then place it in a shallow dish.
2. Sprinkle meat tenderizer over the meat.
3. Whisk rest of the ingredients and spread this marinade over the meat.
4. Marinate the meat for 4 hours in the refrigerator.
5. Bake the meat for 5 minutes per side at 350°F.
6. Slice and serve.

Nutrition: Calories: 184 kcal Total Fat: 8 g Saturated Fat: 0 g Cholesterol: 43 mg Sodium: 208 mg Total Carbs: 3 g

36. Sirloin with Squash and Pineapple

Preparation Time: 10 minutes

Cooking Time: 9 minutes

Servings: 2

Ingredients:

- 8 ounces canned pineapple slices
- 2 garlic cloves, minced
- 2 teaspoons ginger root, minced
- 3 teaspoons olive oil
- 1 pound sirloin tips
- 1 medium zucchini, diced
- 1 medium yellow squash, diced
- 1/2 medium red onion, diced

Directions:

1. Mix pineapple juice with 1 teaspoon olive oil, ginger, and garlic in a Ziplock bag.
2. Add sirloin tips to the pineapple juice marinade and seal the bag.
3. Place the bag in the refrigerator overnight.
4. Preheat oven to 450°F.
5. Layer 2 sheet pans with foil and grease it with 1 teaspoon olive oil.
6. Spread the squash, onion, and pineapple rings in the prepared pans.

7. Bake them for 5 minutes then transfer to the serving plate.
8. Place the marinated sirloin tips on a baking sheet and bake for 4 minutes in the oven.
9. Transfer the sirloin tips to the roasted vegetables.
10. Serve.

Nutrition: Calories: 264 kcal Total Fat: 12 g Saturated Fat: 0 g Cholesterol: 74 mg Sodium: 150 mg Total Carbs: 14 g

37. Slow-Cooked BBQ Beef

Preparation Time: 10 minutes

Cooking Time: 30 minutes

Servings: 4

Ingredients:

- 4-pound pot roast
- 2 cups of water
- ¾ cup ketchup
- 1/4 cup brown sugar
- 1/3 cup vinegar
- 1/2 teaspoon allspice
- 1/4 cup onion

Directions:

1. Add 2 cups water and roast to a Crockpot and cover it.
2. Cook for 10 hours on LOW setting, then drain it while keeping 1 cup of its liquid.
3. Transfer the cooked meat to a 9x13 pan and set it aside.
4. Whisk 1 cup liquid, ketchup, vinegar, brown sugar, minced onion, and allspice in a bowl.
5. Add beef to the marinade and mix well to coat, then marinate overnight in the refrigerator.
6. Spread it on a baking pan then bake for 30 minutes at 350°F.
7. Serve.

Nutrition: Calories: 303 kcal Total Fat: 17 g Saturated Fat: 0 g Cholesterol: 71 mg Sodium: 207 mg Total Carbs: 7 g

38. Lemon Sprouts

Preparation Time: 10 minutes

Cooking Time: 0

Servings: 4

Ingredients:

- 1 pound Brussels sprouts, trimmed and shredded
- 8 tablespoons olive oil
- 1 lemon, juiced and zested
- Salt and pepper to taste
- ¾ cup spicy almond and seed mix

Directions:

1. Take a bowl and mix in lemon juice, salt, pepper and olive oil
2. Mix well
3. Stir in shredded Brussels sprouts and toss
4. Let it sit for 10 minutes
5. Add nuts and toss
6. Serve and enjoy!

Nutrition: Calories: 382 Fat: 36g Carbohydrates: 9g Protein: 7g

39. Lemon and Broccoli Platter

Preparation Time: 10 minutes

Cooking Time: 15 minutes

Servings: 6

Ingredients:

- 2 heads broccoli, separated into florets
- 2 teaspoons extra virgin olive oil
- 1 teaspoon salt
- 1/2 teaspoon black pepper
- 1 garlic clove, minced
- 1/2 teaspoon lemon juice

Directions:

1. Preheat your oven to 400 °F
2. Take a large-sized bowl and add broccoli florets
3. Drizzle olive oil and season with pepper, salt, and garlic
4. Spread the broccoli out in a single even layer on a baking sheet
5. Bake for 15-20 minutes until fork tender
6. Squeeze lemon juice on top
7. Serve and enjoy!

Nutrition: Calories: 49 Fat: 1.9g Carbohydrates: 7g Protein: 3g

40. Chicken Liver Stew

Preparation Time: 10 minutes

Cooking Time: 20 minutes

Servings: 2

Ingredients:

- 10 ounces chicken livers
- 1-ounce onion, chopped
- 2 ounces sour cream
- 1 tablespoon olive oil
- Salt to taste

Directions:

1. Take a pan and place it over medium heat
2. Add oil and let it heat up
3. Add onions and fry until just browned
4. Add livers and season with salt
5. Cook until livers are half cooked
6. Transfer the mix to a stew pot
7. Add sour cream and cook for 20 minutes
8. Serve and enjoy!

Nutrition: Calories: 146 Fat: 9g Carbohydrates: 2g Protein: 15g

41. Simple Lamb Chops

Preparation Time: 35 minutes

Cooking Time: 5 minutes

Servings: 3

Ingredients:

- 1/4 cup olive oil
- 1/4 cup mint, fresh and chopped
- 8 lamb rib chops
- 1 tablespoon garlic, minced
- 1 tablespoon rosemary, fresh and chopped

Directions:

1. Add rosemary, garlic, mint, olive oil into a bowl and mix well
2. Keep a tablespoon of the mixture on the side for later use
3. Toss lamb chops into the marinade, letting them marinate for 30 minutes
4. Take a cast-iron skillet and place it over medium-high heat
5. Add lamb and cook for 2 minutes per side for medium-rare
6. Let the lamb rest for a few minutes and drizzle the remaining marinade
7. Serve and enjoy!

Nutrition: Calories: 566 Fat: 40g Carbohydrates: 2g Protein: 47g

42. Chicken and Mushroom Stew

Preparation Time: 10 minutes

Cooking Time: 35 minutes

Servings: 4

Ingredients:

- 4 chicken breast halves, cut into bite-sized pieces
- 1 pound mushrooms, sliced (5-6 cups)
- 1 bunch spring onion, chopped
- 4 tablespoons olive oil
- 1 teaspoon thyme
- Salt and pepper as needed

Directions:

1. Take a large deep frying pan and place it over medium-high heat
2. Add oil and let it heat up
3. Add chicken and cook for 4-5 minutes per side until slightly browned
4. Add spring onions and mushrooms, season with salt and pepper according to your taste
5. Stir
6. Cover with lid and bring the mix to a boil
7. Lower heat and simmer for 25 minutes
8. Serve!

Nutrition: Calories: 247 Fat: 12g Carbohydrates: 10g Protein: 23g

SNACKS

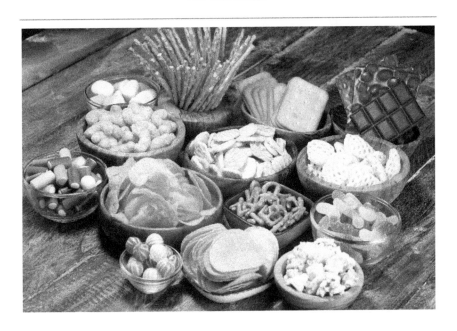

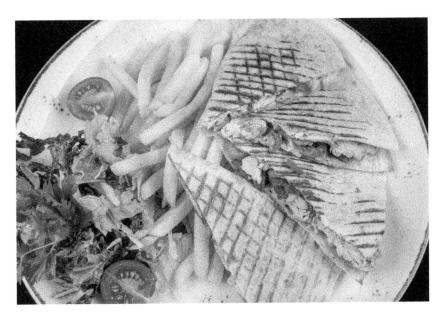

43. Hummus Deviled Eggs

Preparation Time: 10 minutes

Cooking Time: 0 minutes

Servings: 6

Ingredients:

- 6 hard-boiled eggs
- 1/2 cup hummus
- Paprika

Directions:

1. Slice the hardboiled eggs in half lengthwise and remove the yolk.
2. Fill the egg whites with hummus and sprinkle with paprika before serving.

Nutrition: Calories: 179 kcal Protein: 11.03 g Fat: 12.41 g Carbohydrates: 5.14 g

44. Hummus with Celery

Preparation Time: 15 minutes

Cooking Time: 0 minutes

Servings: 4

Ingredients:

- 1/4 cup lemon juice
- 1/4 cup tahini
- 3 cloves of garlic, crushed
- 2 tablespoons extra virgin olive oil
- 1/2 teaspoon salt
- 1/2 teaspoon cumin
- 1 (15-ounce) can chickpeas
- 2 to 3 tablespoons water
- Dash of paprika
- 6 stalks celery, cut into 2-inch pieces
- 3 tablespoons salsa

Directions:

1. Using a food processor mix the lemon juice and tahini for about a minute, until it is smooth. Scrape the sides down and process for 30 more seconds.
2. Add the garlic, olive oil, salt, and cumin. Blend for about 1 minute.
3. Drain the chickpeas, put the half of them on the food processor, and blend for another minute. Scrape down the

sides, add the other half of the chickpeas, and process until smooth, about 2 minutes. If it like a little too thick, add water, 1 tablespoon at a time until you reach the desired consistency.
4. Fill the celery sticks with hummus and sprinkle paprika on top.
5. Serve with salsa for dipping.

Nutrition: Calories: 240 kcal   Protein: 9.27 g   Fat: 14.51 g   Carbohydrates: 21.01 g

45. Lemony Ginger Cookies

Preparation Time: 15 minutes + 30 minutes chill time

Cooking Time: 10-12 minutes

Servings: 25

Ingredients:

- 1/2 cup arrowroot flour
- 1 1/2 cups stevia
- 3/4 teaspoon salt
- 1/2 teaspoon baking soda
- 1 teaspoon nutritional yeast
- 3 inches of ginger root, peeled and diced
- 1 1/2 cup coconut butter, softened
- Zest of 1 lemon
- 2 teaspoons vanilla

Directions:

1. Set the oven to 350F, then line two or three cookie sheets with parchment paper.
2. Mix the arrowroot flour, stevia, salt, soda, and yeast in a bowl.
3. In another bowl, put the remaining ingredients and mix well.
4. Put in the dry ingredients gradually until well combined. If the dough is too soft, put an additional 1 to 2 tablespoons of arrowroot powder. The dough will stiffen when chilled, so be careful.

5. Wrap the dough in parchment and press it flat. Chill for 30 minutes.
6. Take a chunk of the chilled dough and flatten it between two pieces of parchment until it is 1/8 inch thick. Dust with a little arrowroot powder and cut into shapes.
7. Place on baking sheets about 1 inch apart and bake 10 to 12 minutes. Cool on cookie sheets for 15 minutes before removing.

Nutrition: Calories: 112 kcal Protein: 0.44 g Fat: 11.3 g Carbohydrates: 2.49 g

46. Mandarin Cottage Cheese

Preparation Time: 5 minutes

Cooking Time: 0 minutes

Servings: 1

Ingredients:

- 1/2 cup low-fat cottage cheese
- 1/2 cup canned mandarin mangos
- 1 1/2 tablespoons slivered almonds

Directions:

1. Place the cottage cheese in a bowl.
2. Drain the mandarin mangos, place them atop the cottage cheese, and sprinkle with almonds.

Nutrition: Calories: 360 kcal Protein: 26.24 g Fat: 21.37 g Carbohydrates: 15.22 g

47. Mushroom Chips

Preparation Time: 10 minutes

Cooking Time: 45-60 minutes

Servings: 2-4

Ingredients:

- 16 ounces of king oyster mushrooms
- 2 tablespoons ghee
- Kosher salt and ground pepper to taste

Directions:

1. Set the oven to 300F, then line two cookie sheets with parchment paper.
2. Cut every mushroom in half lengthwise, then cut with a mandolin into 1/8 inch slices or strips. Place them on cookie sheets with some room in between. Melt the ghee and brush it over the mushrooms, then season with the salt and pepper.
3. Bake for at least 45 minutes to 1 hour, until they are completely crisp. Store in airtight containers.

Nutrition: Calories: 62 kcal Protein: 5.58 g Fat: 2 g Carbohydrates: 7.97 g

DESSERTS

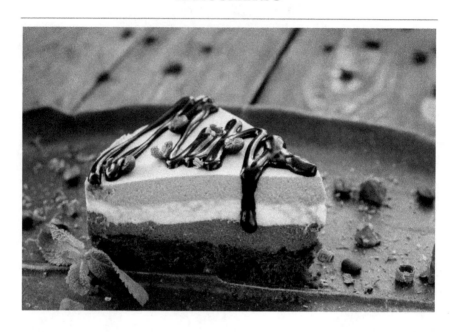

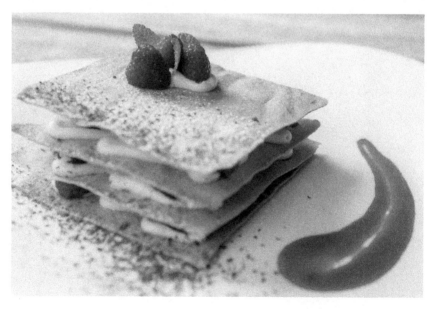

48. Pound Cake with Pineapple

Preparation Time: 10 minutes

Cooking Time: 50 minutes

Servings: 24

Ingredients

- 3 cups of all-purpose flour, sifted
- 3 cups of sugar
- 1 ½ cups of butter
- 6 whole eggs and 3 egg whites
- 1 teaspoon of vanilla extract
- 1 10. ounce can of pineapple chunks, rinsed and crushed (keep juice aside).
- For glaze:
- 1 cup of sugar
- 1 stick of unsalted butter or margarine
- Reserved juice from the pineapple

Directions

1. Preheat the oven at 350F/180C.
2. Beat the sugar and the butter with a hand mixer until creamy and smooth.
3. Slowly add the eggs (one or two every time) and stir well after pouring each egg.
4. Add the vanilla extract, follow up with the flour and stir well.
5. Add the drained and chopped pineapple.

6. Pour the mixture into a greased cake tin and bake for 45-50 minutes.
7. In a small saucepan, combine the sugar with the butter and pineapple juice. Stir every few seconds and bring to boil. Cook until you get a creamy to thick glaze consistency.
8. Pour the glaze over the cake while still hot.
9. Let cook for at least 10 seconds and serve.

Nutrition: Calories: 407.4 kcal Carbohydrate: 79 g Protein: 4.25 g Sodium: 118.97 mg Potassium: 180.32 mg Phosphorus: 66.37 mg Dietary Fiber: 2.25 g Fat: 16.48 g

49. Apple Crunch Pie

Preparation Time: 10 minutes

Cooking Time: 35 minutes

Servings: 8

Ingredients

- 4 large tart apples, peeled, seeded and sliced
- ½ cup of white all-purpose flour
- ⅓ cup margarine
- 1 cup of sugar
- ¾ cup of rolled oat flakes
- ½ teaspoon of ground nutmeg

Directions

1. Preheat the oven to 375F/180C.
2. Place the apples over a lightly greased square pan (around 7 inches).
3. Mix the rest of the ingredients in a medium bowl with and spread the batter over the apples.
4. Bake for 30-35 minutes or until the top crust has gotten golden brown.
5. Serve hot.

Nutrition: Calories: 261.9 kcal Carbohydrate: 47.2 g Protein: 1.5 g Sodium: 81 mg Potassium: 123.74 mg Phosphorus: 35.27 mg Dietary Fiber: 2.81 g Fat: 7.99 g

50. Vanilla Custard

Preparation Time: 7 minutes

Cooking Time: 10 minutes

Servings: 10

Ingredients

- Egg – 1
- Vanilla – 1/8 Teaspoon
- Nutmeg – 1/8 Teaspoon
- Almond Almond Milk – ½ Cup
- Stevia - 2 Tablespoon

Directions

1. Scald The Almond Milk Then Let It Cool Slightly.
2. Break The Egg Into A Bowl And Beat It With The Nutmeg.
3. Add The Scalded Almond Milk, The Vanilla, And The Sweetener To Taste. Mix Well.
4. Place The Bowl In A Baking Pan Filled With ½ Deep Of Water.
5. Bake For 30 Minutes At 325F.
6. Serve.

Nutrition: Calories: 167.3 Fat: 9g Carb: 11g Phosphorus: 205mg Potassium: 249mg Sodium: 124mg Protein: 10g

51. Chocolate Chip Cookies

Preparation Time: 7 minutes

Cooking Time: 10 minutes

Servings: 10

Ingredients

- Semi-sweet chocolate chips – ½ cup
- Baking soda – ½ teaspoon
- Vanilla – ½ teaspoon
- Egg – 1
- Flour – 1 cup
- Margarine – ½ cup
- Stevia – 4 teaspoons

Directions

1. Sift the dry ingredients.
2. Cream the margarine, stevia, vanilla and egg with a whisk.
3. Add flour mixture and beat well.
4. Stir in the chocolate chips, then drop teaspoonsful of the mixture over a greased baking sheet.
5. Bake the cookies for about 10 minutes at 375F.
6. Cool and serve.

Nutrition: Calories: 106.2 Fat: 7g Carb: 8.9g Phosphorus: 19mg Potassium: 28mg Sodium: 98mg Protein: 1.5g